Pebble® Plus

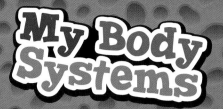

My Body Systems

My Skeletal System

A 4D Book

by Martha E. H. Rustad

Consultant:
Natasha Kasbekar, M.D., Pediatrician
Kids Health Partners, LLC, Skokie, Ill.

PEBBLE
a capstone imprint

Download the Capstone 4D app!

- Ask an adult to download the Capstone 4D app.
- Scan the cover and stars inside the book for additional content.

When you scan a spread, you'll find fun extra stuff to go with this book! You can also find these things on the web at www.capstone4D.com using the password: bones.00191

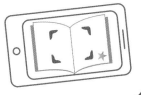

Pebble Plus is published by Pebble
1710 Roe Crest Drive, North Mankato, Minnesota 56003
www.mycapstone.com

Library of Congress Cataloging-in-Publication Data
Names: Rustad, Martha E. H. (Martha Elizabeth Hillman), 1975– author.
Title: My skeletal system : a 4D book / by Martha E. H. Rustad.
Description: North Mankato, Minnesota : Pebble, [2019] | Series: Pebble Plus. My body systems | Audience: Age 4–8.
Identifiers: LCCN 2018004146 (print) | LCCN 2018004312 (ebook) | ISBN 9781977100276 (eBook PDF) | ISBN 9781977100191 (hardcover) | ISBN 9781977100238 (paperback)
Subjects: LCSH: Musculoskeletal system—Juvenile literature. | Human locomotion—Juvenile literature.
Classification: LCC QP301 (ebook) | LCC QP301 .R87 2019 (print) | DDC 612.7—dc23
LC record available at https://lccn.loc.gov/2018004146

Editorial Credits
Emily Raij, editor; Charmaine Whitman, designer; Morgan Walters, media researcher; Laura Manthe, production specialist

Image Credits
iStockphoto: Studio1One, 13; Shutterstock: altanaka, (girl) Cover, Blend Images, 19, Denis Kuvaev, 1, Designua, 11, eranicle, (inset) Cover, Jemastock, (leg bone) Cover, Kiselev Andrey Valerevich, 5, Meilun, 7, MSSA, design element throughout, nehophoto, 21, Pretty Vectors, left 17, sciencepics, 9, Sebastian Kaulitzki, 15, struna, right 17, yodiyim, 11

Printed and bound in the United States.
PA017

Note to Parents and Teachers

The My Body Systems set supports the national science standards related to structures and processes. This book describes and illustrates the skeletal system. The images support early readers in understanding the text. The repetition of words and phrases helps early readers learn new words. This book also introduces early readers to subject-specific vocabulary words, which are defined in the Glossary section. Early readers may need assistance to read some words and to use the Table of Contents, Glossary, Read More, Internet Sites, Critical Thinking Questions, and Index sections of the book.

Table of Contents

Skeletons and Bones

Boo! Did I scare you?

My skeleton is made of bones.

They hold up my body.

Without bones I would be

a blob. That's scary!

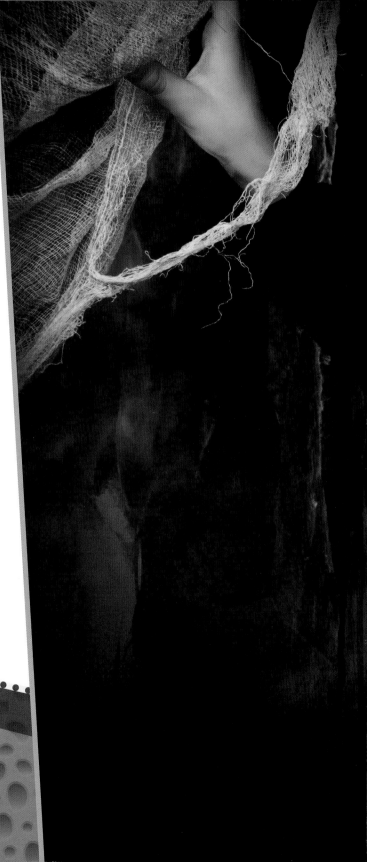

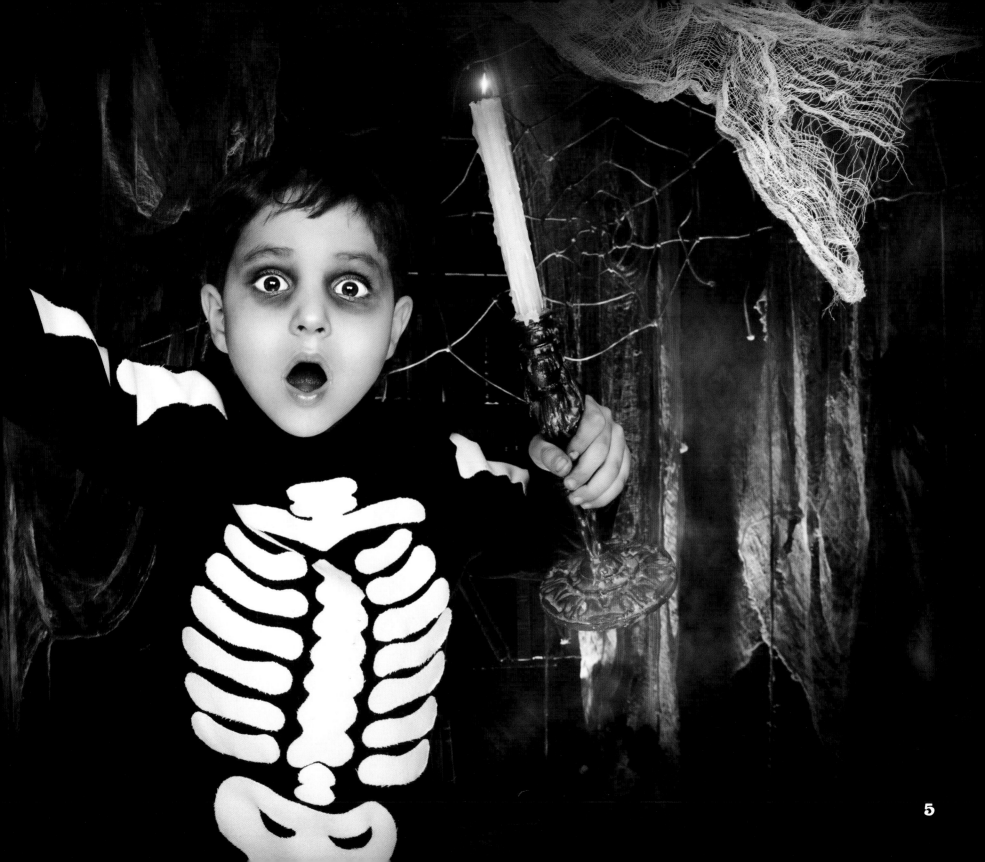

Bones are hard on the outside.

They protect my organs.

My rib cage keeps my heart

and lungs safe. A hard skull

protects my brain.

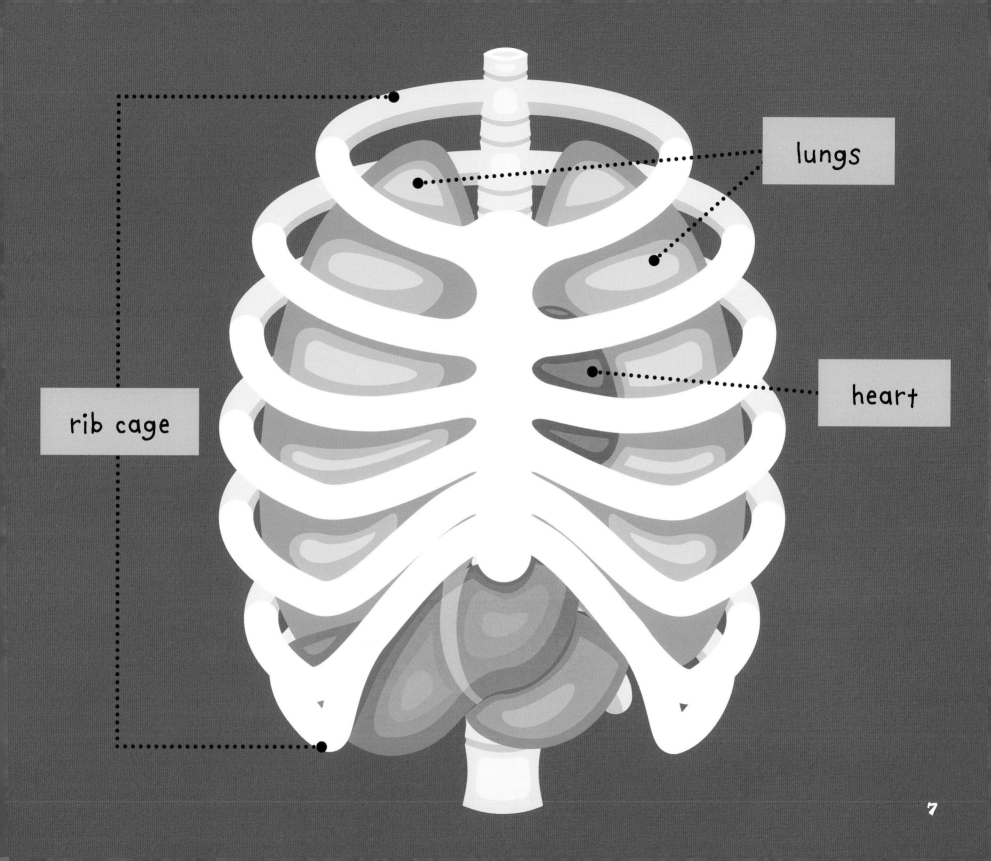

lungs

rib cage

heart

Parts of a Skeleton

My bones have a thin covering. Blood vessels and nerves are in this layer. Blood moves through the vessels. It gives nutrients to bones.

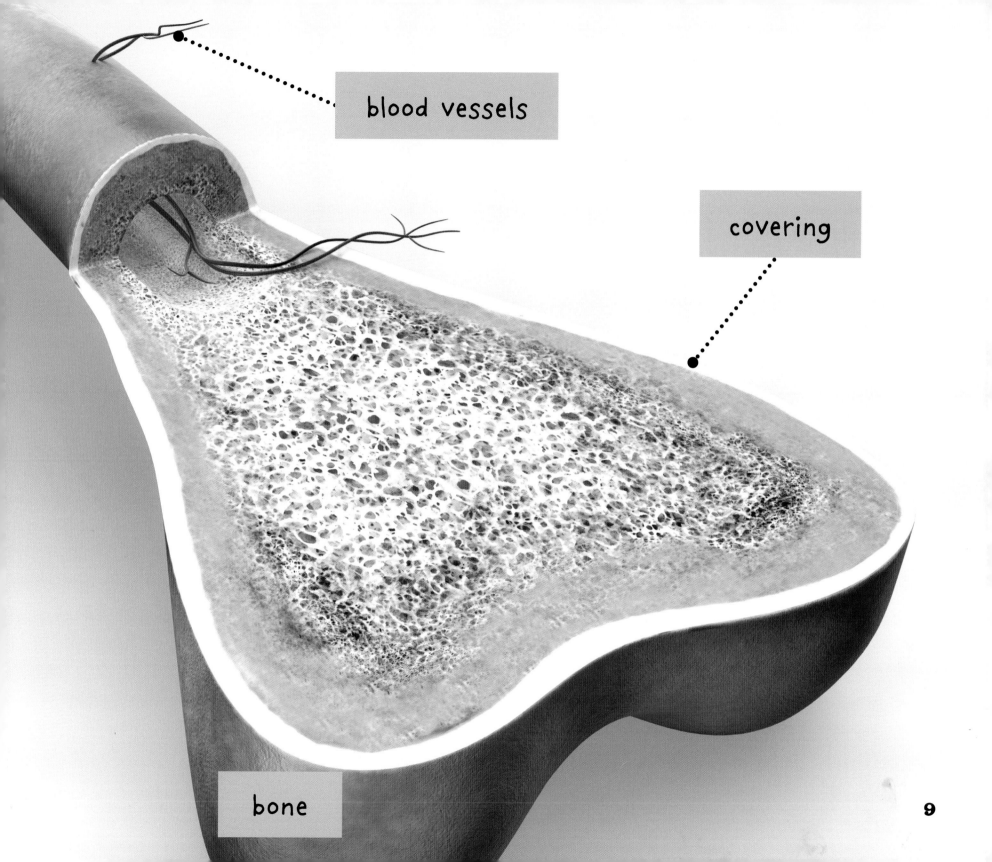

blood vessels

covering

bone

9

Soft marrow fills my bones.

It makes blood cells.

Blood vessels carry the cells

around my body.

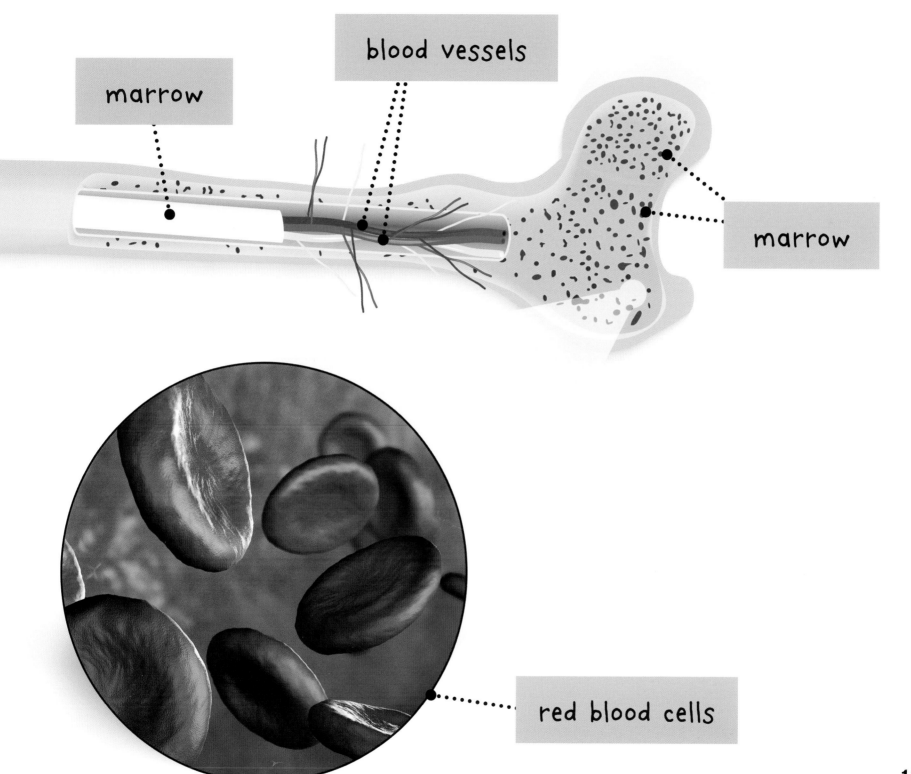

marrow

blood vessels

marrow

red blood cells

Two bones meet at a joint.

Joints help me move.

One joint moves my knee back
and forth. Another joint moves
my shoulder in circles.

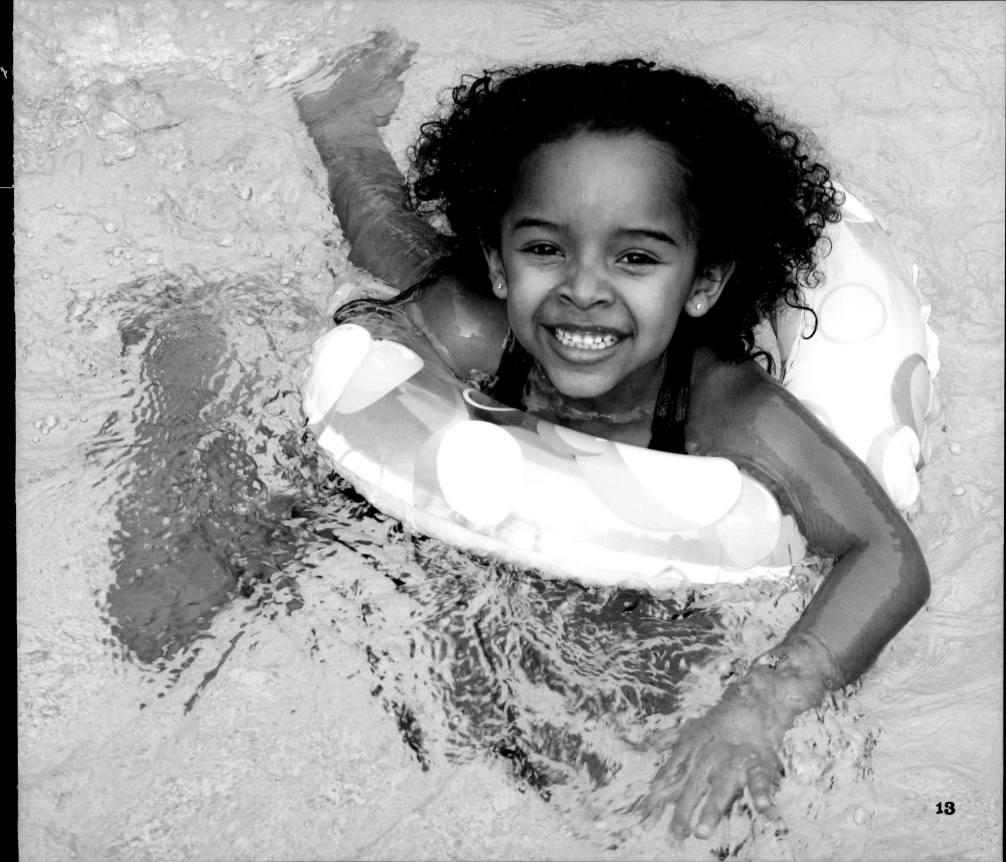

My spine runs up my back.

Inside is my spinal cord.

It holds a group of nerves.

Nerves send information

to my brain.

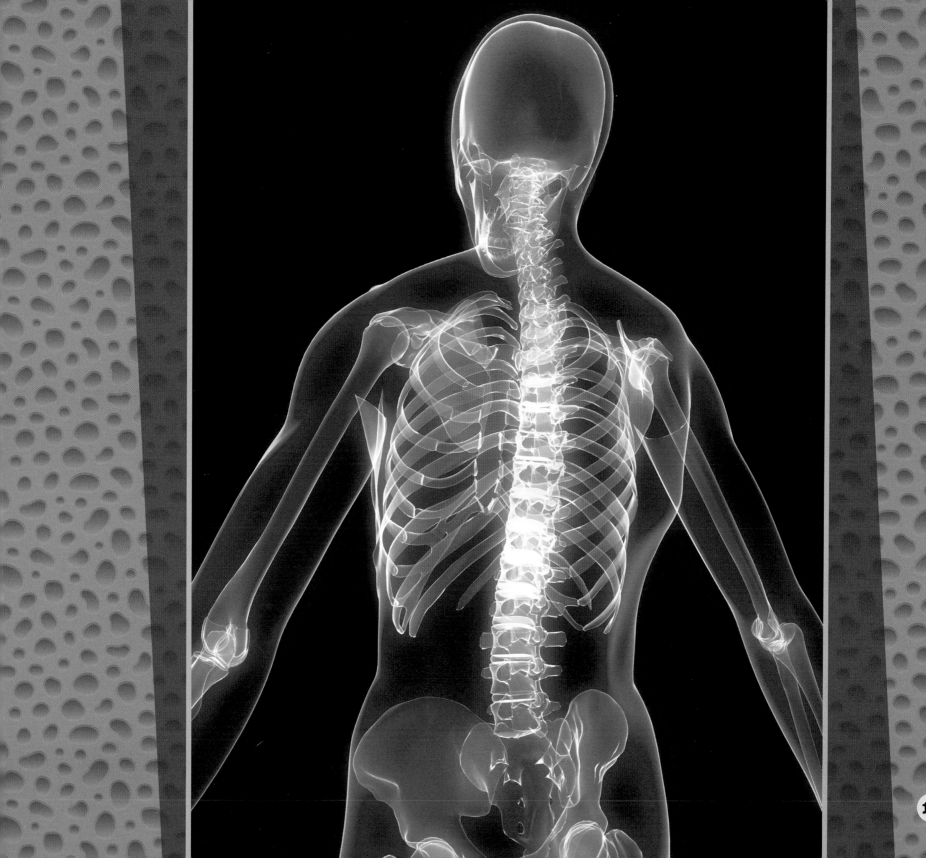

15

The femur is my largest bone.

It moves my leg when I run.

The stapes is my smallest bone.

It helps me hear.

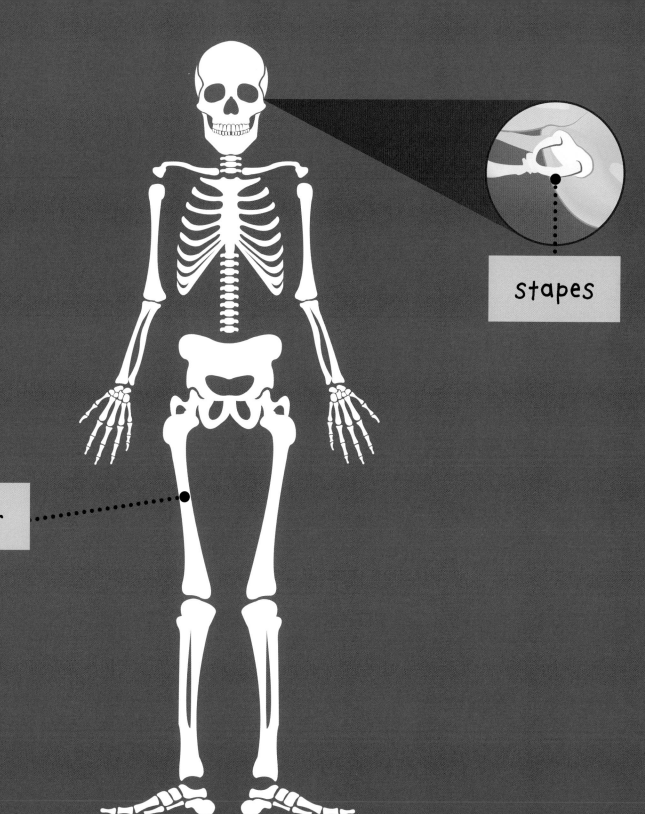

stapes

femur

Keeping Bones Healthy

Snap! Ouch!

My bones can break.

Bones fix themselves. A doctor makes sure they are lined up.

Bones take many weeks to heal.

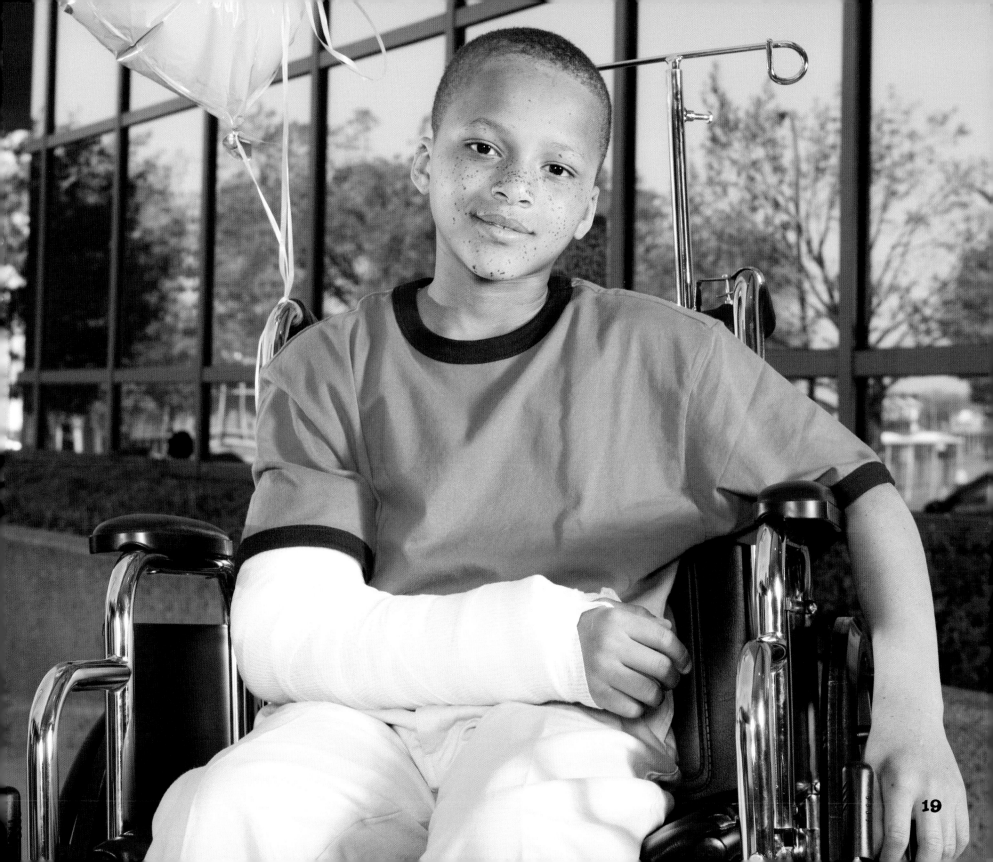

I eat healthy foods.
They have vitamins that keep
my bones strong. I help
my bones so they can help me.
Bodies need bones!

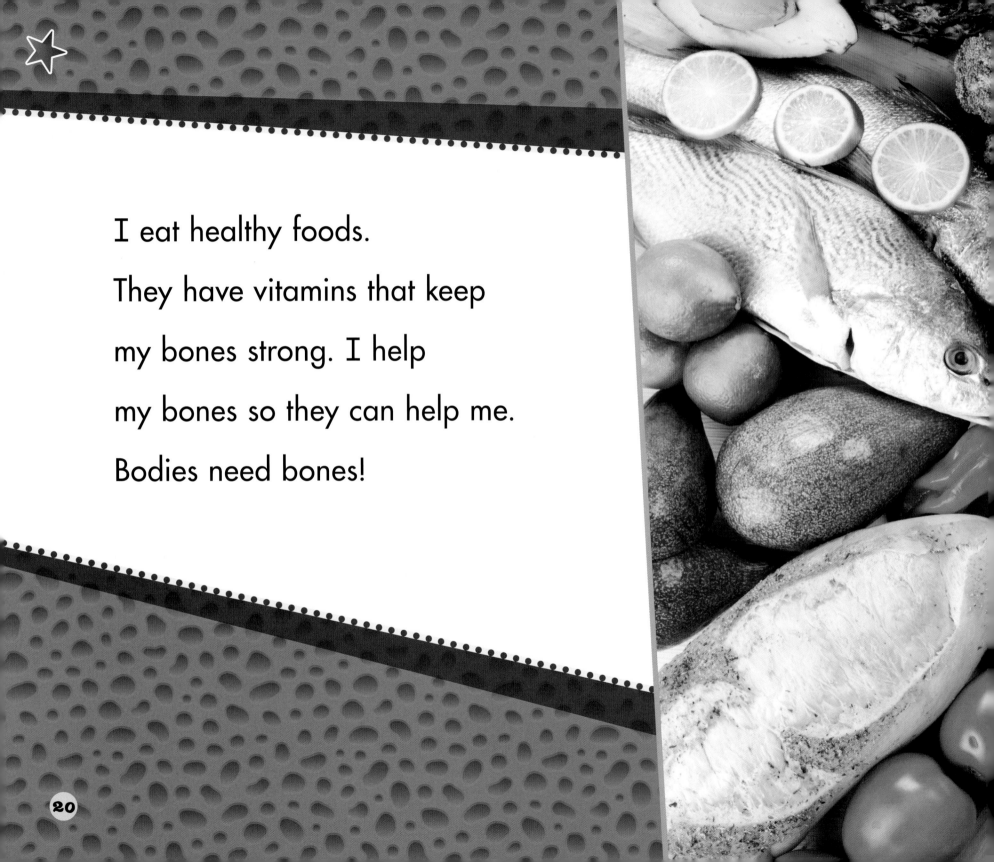

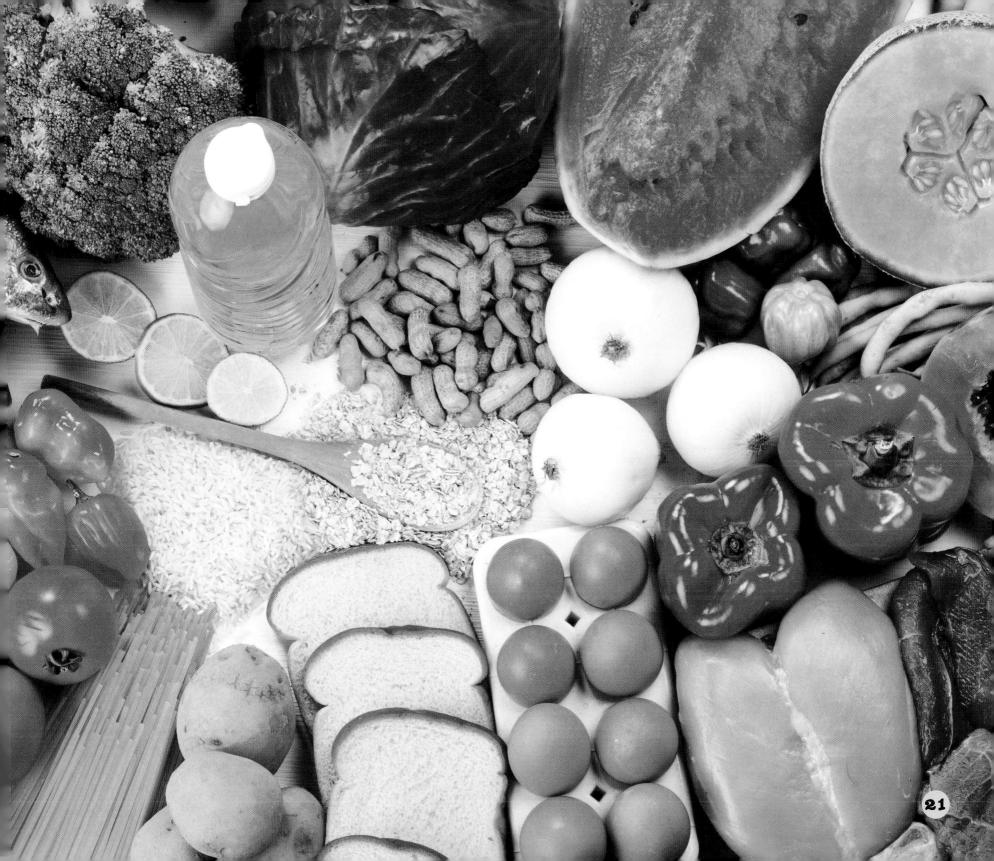

Glossary

blood cell—the smallest part of the blood

blood vessel—a narrow tube that carries blood through your body

femur—thigh bone

joint—the place where two bones meet; knees, elbows, hips, and shoulders are joints.

marrow—the soft material inside bones that is used to make blood cells

nerves—stringy bands of tissue that connect and carry signals from different body parts to the brain

nutrient—something that is needed by people, animals, and plants to stay healthy and strong

organ—a body part that does a certain job

skull—the set of bones in the head; the skull protects the brain, eyes, and inner ears.

stapes—small, inner ear bone

vitamin—a nutrient that helps keep people healthy

Read More

Bassington, Cyril. *Your Bones*. Know Your Body. New York: Gareth Stevens Publishing, 2016.

Brett, Flora. *Your Skeletal System Works!* Your Body Systems. North Mankato, Minn.: Capstone Press, 2015.

Winston, Robert. *The Skeleton Book*. New York: DK Publishing, 2016.

Internet Sites

Use FactHound to find Internet sites related to this book.

Visit *www.facthound.com*

Just type in 9781977100191 and go.

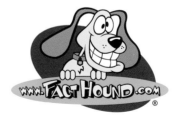

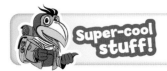
Check out projects, games and lots more at
www.capstonekids.com

Critical Thinking Questions

1. How do bones protect organs?

2. How do bones move?

3. How can you keep your bones strong and healthy?

Index